Pediatric intensive care algorithms
Nemba ICU

Maria Inguanzo Ortiz

December 2022

Pediatric intensive care algorithms
Maria Inguanzo Ortiz

Copyright© 2022 by Maria Inguanzo Ortiz

All rights reserved. This book or any portion thereof may not be reproduced or used in any manner whatsoever without the express written permission of the author except for the use of brief quotations in a book review or scholarly journal.

First printing: 2023

ISBN 978-1-4478-4718-2

Index

Normal vital signs 5
Pediatric vital signs reference chart 7
Warning signs 8
    Pediatric Early Warning Score PEWS 8
    PEWS score calculation and intervention 9
Scores and scales 10
    Asthma score 10
    Glasgow coma score 11
    AVPU score 12
Pediatric initial Assessment 13
ABCDE approach 14
Airway 16
    Assess airway 16
    Position 16
    Open airway maneuvers 16
    Oropharyngeal airway 18
    Endotracheal tube (ETT) 19
Breathing 21
    Assessment 21
    Recognizing respiratory problems 22
    Bag mask ventilation 23
    Respiratory failure: initial management 25
    Respiratory emergencies flowchart 26
Circulation 27
    Assess Circulation 27
    Recognizing shock 27
    Shock management 28
    Pediatric septic Shock algorithm 29
    Pediatric cardiac arrest algorithm 30
Fluid therapy 31
    Assessment 31
    Fluid therapy: Why? What? How much? 31

- Fluid therapy flowchart 34
- Maintenance fluid calculator 34
- Newborn fluid therapy 35

Disability
- Assess disability 36
- Glasgow coma scale 36
- Blood glucose test 37
- Abnormal pupil responses and possible causes 37
- Seizures flowchart 38

Bibliography 39

Normal vital signs

Normal Heart Rates*

Age	Awake rate (beats/min)	Sleeping rate (beats/min)
Neonate	100-205	90-160
Infant	100-180	90-160
Toddler	98-140	80-120
Preschooler	80-120	65-100
School-age child	75-118	58-90
Adolescent	60-100	50-90

*Always consider the patient's normal range and clinical condition. Heart rate will normally increase with fever or stress.

Illustration 1 Normal heart rate, AHA, 2020

Normal Respiratory Rates*

Age	Rate (breaths/min)
Infant	30-53
Toddler	22-37
Preschooler	20-28
School-age child	18-25
Adolescent	12-20

*Consider the patient's normal range. The child's respiratory rate is expected to increase in the presence of fever or stress.
Data from Fleming S et al. *Lancet*. 2011;377(9770):1011-1018.

Illustration 2 Normal respiratory rate, AHA, 2020

Normal Blood Pressures

Age	Systolic pressure (mm Hg)*	Diastolic pressure (mm Hg)*	Mean arterial pressure (mm Hg)†
Birth (12 h, <1000 g)	39-59	16-36	28-42‡
Birth (12 h, 3 kg)	60-76	31-45	48-57
Neonate (96 h)	67-84	35-53	45-60
Infant (1-12 mo)	72-104	37-56	50-62
Toddler (1-2 y)	86-106	42-63	49-62
Preschooler (3-5 y)	89-112	46-72	58-69
School-age child (6-9 y)	97-115	57-76	66-72
Preadolescent (10-12 y)	102-120	61-80	71-79
Adolescent (12-15 y)	110-131	64-83	73-84

*Systolic and diastolic blood pressure ranges assume 50th percentile for height for children 1 year and older.
†Mean arterial pressures (diastolic pressure + [difference between systolic and diastolic pressure ÷ 3]) for 1 year and older, assuming 50th percentile for height.
‡Approximately equal to postconception age in weeks (may add 5 mm Hg).

Illustration 3 Normal blood pressure, AHA, 2020

Normal oxygenation:

	Oxygenation status	Action
Sa02 95-100%	**Normal**	Routine care
Sa02 92-94%	Almost normal	Monitoring
Sat 90-92%	Hypoxemia (mild)	Monitoring Consider oxygen
Sa02 80-89%	Hypoxemia (moderate)	Monitoring Give oxygen! ABCD
Sa02 < 80%	Hypoxemia (severe)	Monitoring Give oxygen! ABCD
Goal when giving oxygen → Sa02 95-97%		

Pediatric vital signs reference chart

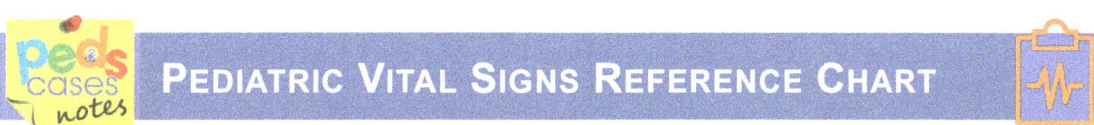

Illustration 4 Pedscases: pediatric vital signs reference chart, The Hospital for Sick Children in Toronto, Canada.

PICU algorithms　　　　　　　　　　　　　　　　　　　　　　　　　Nemba ICU

Warning signs

Pediatric Early Warning Score PEWS

- PEWS is a tool to aid recognition of sick and deteriorating children
- PEWS should be calculated every time observations are recorded

0-11 months	3	1	0	1	3
Heart rate	≤99	100-109	110-160	161-169	≥170
Blood pressure	≤59	60-69	70-100	101-109	≥110
Capillary refill			< 2 sec	2-4 sec	>4 sec
Resp rate	≤19	20-29	30-50	51-69	≥70
SaO2	≤91	92-93	≥94		
O2 delivery			air	O2	
Temperature	≤ 34,9	35-35,9	36-37,9	≥38	
Conscious	P/U	V/sleeping	Alert, playing		

12-23 months	3	1	0	1	3
Heart rate	≤79	80-89	100-150	151-159	≥160
Blood pressure	≤59	60-69	70-100	101-109	≥110
Capillary refill			< 2 sec	2-4 sec	>4 sec
Resp rate	≤19	20-24	25-40	41-59	≥60
SaO2	≤91	92-93	≥94		
O2 delivery			air	O2	
Temperature	≤ 34,9	35-35,9	36-37,9	≥38	
Conscious	P/U	V/sleeping	Alert, playing		

2-4 years	3	1	0	1	3
Heart rate	≤69	70-89	90-139	140-149	≥150
Blood pressure	≤69	70-79	80-100	101-119	≥120
Capillary refill			< 2 sec	2-4 sec	>4 sec
Resp rate	≤14	15-19	20-24	35-49	≥50
SaO2	≤91	92-93	≥94		
O2 delivery			air	O2	
Temperature	≤ 34,9	35-35,9	36-37,9	≥38	
Conscious	P/U	V/sleeping	Alert, playing		

5-11 years	3	1	0	1	3
Heart rate	≤59	60-79	80-129	130-139	≥140
Blood pressure	≤79	80-89	90-109	110-129	≥130
Capillary refill			< 2 sec	2-4 sec	>4 sec
Resp rate	≤14	15-19	20-29	30-39	≥40
SaO2	≤91	92-93	≥94		
O2 delivery			air	O2	
Temperature	≤ 34,9	35-35,9	36-37,9	≥38	
Conscious (AVPU)	P/U	V/sleeping	Alert/playing		

>12 years	3	1	0	1	3
Heart rate	≤49	50-69	70-109	110-129	≥130
Blood pressure	≤89	90-99	100-119	120-139	≥140
Capillary refill			< 2 sec	2-4 sec	>4 sec
Resp rate	≤9	10-14	15-24	25-34	≥35
SaO2	≤91	92-93	≥94		
O2 delivery			air	O2	
Temperature	≤ 34,9	35-35,9	36-37,9	≥38	
Conscious	P/U	V/sleeping	Alert/playing		

PEWS score calculation and intervention

Score	Monitorization	Location	Response
0-1	4 hourly	Routine protocol	Routine
2	2-4 hourly	Routine protocol	Routine
3	1 hourly	Alert ICU	ABCD (page 12)
4-5	continous	ICU	ABCD (page 12)
6	continous	ICU	ABCD (page 12)
≥7	continous	ICU	ABCD (page 12)

Scores and scales

Asthma score

Table 34. Classifying Mild, Moderate, and Severe Asthma

Parameter*	Mild	Moderate	Severe	Respiratory arrest imminent
Breathless	Walking Can lie down	Talking (Infant will have softer, shorter cry; difficulty feeding) Prefers sitting	At rest (Infant will stop feeding) Hunched forward	
Talks in	Sentences	Phrases	Words	
Alertness	May be agitated	Usually agitated	Usually agitated	Drowsy or confused
Respiratory rate†	Increased	Increased	Often >30/min	
Accessory muscles and suprasternal retractions	Usually not	Usually	Usually	Paradoxical thoracoabdominal movement
Wheeze	Moderate, often only end-expiration	Loud	Usually loud	Absence of wheeze
Pulse/min‡	<100	100-120	>120	Bradycardia
Pulsus paradoxus	Absent <10 mm Hg	May be present 10-25 mm Hg	Often present >25 mm Hg (adult) 25-40 mm Hg (child)	Absence suggests respiratory muscle fatigue
PEF (if used in clinical practice) after initial bronchodilator % predicted or % personal best	>80%	Approximately 60%-80%	<60% predicted or personal best (<100 L/min adults) or response lasts <2 hours	
PaCO$_2$	Normal, test usually not necessary <45 mm Hg	>60 mm Hg <45 mm Hg	<60 mm Hg; possible cyanosis >45 mm Hg; possible respiratory failure	
SpO$_2$ (room air)%	>95%	91%-95%	<90%	

*The presence of several parameters, but not necessarily all, indicates the general classification of the attack.
†Guide to limits of normal respiratory rate in infants and children: age <2 months, respiratory rate <60/min; age 2-12 months, respiratory rate <50/min; age 1-5 years, respiratory rate <40/min; age 6-8 years, respiratory rate <30/min.
‡Guide to limits of normal pulse rate in infants and children: infant (2-12 months), pulse rate <160/min; toddler (1-2 years), pulse rate <120/min; preschool/school age (2-8 years), pulse rate <110/min.
Adapted from National Heart, Lung, and Blood Institute and World Health Organization. *Global Strategy for Asthma Management and Prevention NHLBI/WHO Workshop Report.* US Department of Health and Human Services; 1997. Publication 97-4051.

Illustration 5 Asthma score, AHA, 2020

Glasgow coma score

Score	Child	Infant
Eye opening		
4	Spontaneously	Spontaneously
3	To verbal command	To shout, speech
2	To pain	To pain
1	No response	No response
Best motor response		
6	Obeys commands	Spontaneous movements
5	Localizes pain	Withdraws to touch
4	Flexion-appropriate withdraw	Flexion-appropriate withdraw
3	Flexion-abnormal (decorticate rigidity)	Flexion-abnormal (decorticate rigidity)
2	Extension (decerebrate rigidity)	Extension (decerebrate rigidity)
1	No response	No response
Best verbal response		
5	Oriented and converses	Smiles, coos, and babbles
4	Disoriented, confused	Cries but is consolable
3	Inappropriate words	Persistent, inappropriate crying and/or screaming
2	Incomprehensible sounds	Moans, grunts to pain
1	No response	No response
Total = 3 to 15		

*Score is the sum of the individual scores from eye opening, best motor response, and best verbal response, using age-specific criteria. GCS score of 13 to 15 indicates mild head injury; GCS score of 9 to 12 indicates moderate head injury; and GCS score of ≤8 indicates severe head injury.

Modified from James HE, Trauner DA. The Glasgow Coma Score and Modified Coma Score for Infants. In: James HE, Anas NG, Perkin RM, eds. *Brain Insults in Infants and Children: Pathophysiology and Management.* Grune & Stratton Inc; 1985:179-182, copyright Elsevier.

Illustration 6 Glasgow coma score, AHA, 2020

AVPU score

- Use AVPU to rapidly evaluate cerebral cortex: level of consciousness

AVPU Pediatric Response Scale:		
A	Alert	The child is awake, active, and appropriately responsive to caregivers and external stimuli
V	Voice	The child responds only to voice (e.g., calling the child's name or speaking loudly).
P	Pain	The child responds only to a painful stimulus, such as a sternal rub or pinching the trapezius
U	Unresponsive	The child does not respond to any stimulus

Pediatric initial Assessment

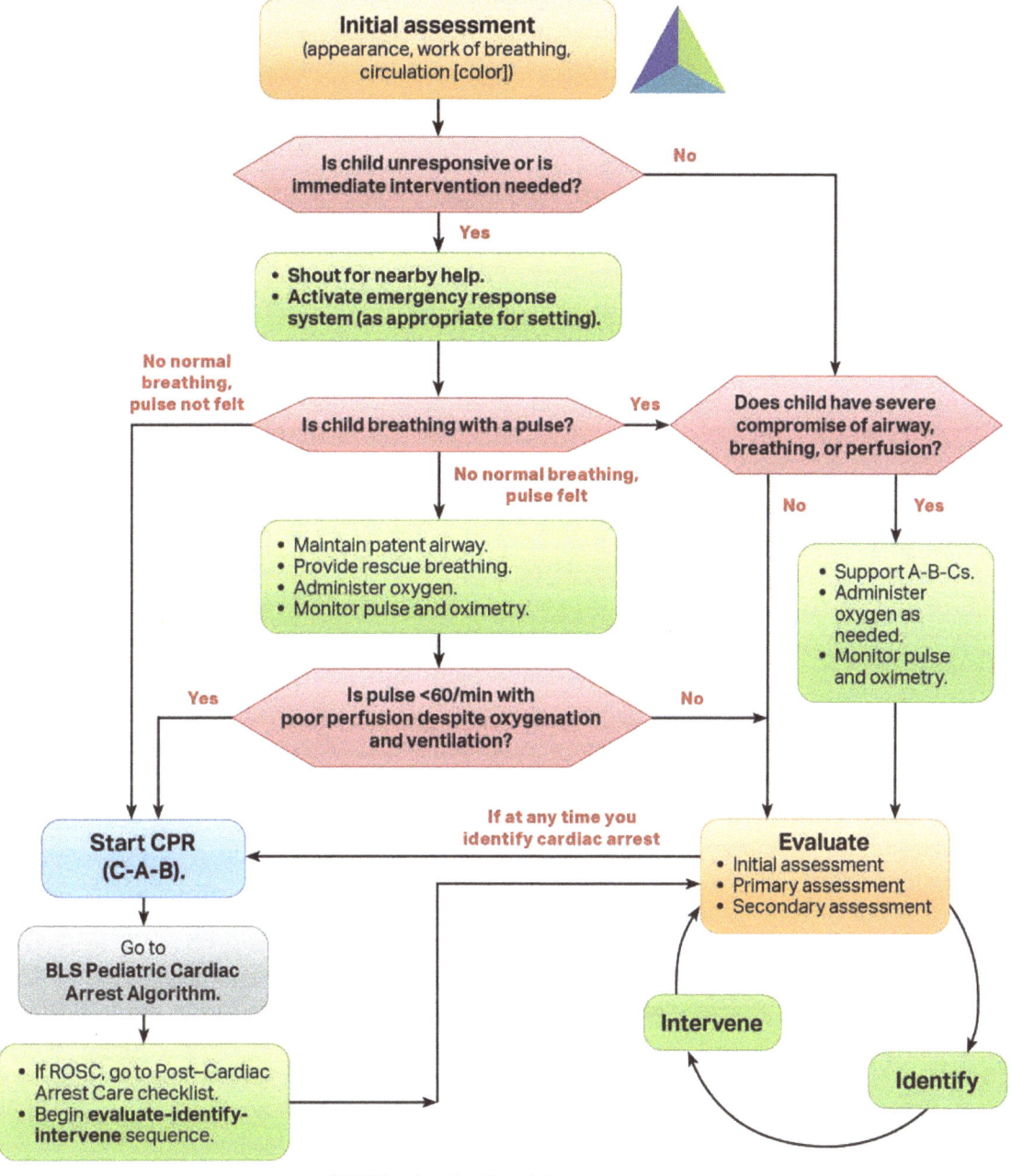

Illustration 7 PALS systematic approach algorithm, AHA; 2020

PICU algorithms 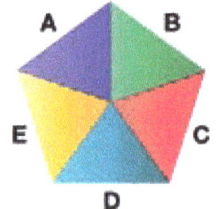 Nemba ICU

ABCDE approach

Evaluate	Situation	Intervention
Airway: Look, listen, feel	Airway open	Allow the child to assume a position of comfort or elevate the head of the bed or Fowler or semi-Fowler position
	Airway not maintainable	Head Tilt-Chin Lift (sniffing position child, neutral infant) or Jaw thrust (page 14)
	Secretions, blood	Suctioning nose and oropharynx
	To improve airway patency	Consider airway adjuncts (OPA) to improve patency (page 16)
Breathing: RR, respiratory pattern, chest expansion, lung sounds		Monitor O2 saturation by pulse oximetry
	SaO2 < 90%	Give oxygen Consider CPAP
	Difficult breathing (retractions, nasal flaring, grunting, head bobbing)	Consider inhaled medication
	No breathing, gasping	Bag-mask ventilation with oxygen (page 21)
		Advanced airway if indicated (page 18)
Circulation: HR, BP, pulses, capillary refill time, skin color and temperature, urine output, level consciousness		Monitor heart rate, ECG rhythm, BP
		Establish vascular access (IV, IO)
	Shock (tachycardia, capillary refill > 2 seconds, ↓ pulses, Discrepancy central vs. Distal pulses, ↓	20 ml/kg Normal Saline 0,9% bolus (x2-3)

	mental status, ↓ urine output, metabolic acidosis (lactic) *Hypotension is a late sign	
	HR < 60 bpm with cardiorespiratory compromise	Start chest compressions 15:2
	Bleeding	Control external bleeding Red blood cell transfusion
Disability: Glasgow coma scale, AVPU, pupils, blood glucose		
	Glucose < 60 mg/dl	Dx10% 2 ml/kg or Dx 50% 0,5 ml/kg
	Brain injury	
	Seizures	ABCD (page 36) Benzodiazepine
Exposure		Temperature
		Assess child fully
	Hypothermia	Correct hypothermia
	Fever	Paracetamol
	Rash, petechiae. purpura	Consider sepsis
	Pain	Painkillers

Airway

Assess airway
- Look for chest or abdomen movement
- Listen for air movement and breath sounds
- Feel for air movement at the nose and mouth

Position

- Fowler:
    - Patient sits upright at an angle between 45 and 60 degrees.
    - The legs of the patient are either bent at the knees or laid out straight on the bed.
    - The position is preferred as an option to combat respiratory distress syndrome since it allows for better chest expansion and improves breathing by facilitating oxygenation.

- Semi-Fowler:
    - Similar to the standard Fowler's position, however, the head and back rest at a lower angle
    - The bed is typically inclined at an angle of 15 to 45 degrees, although 30 degrees is most frequently used

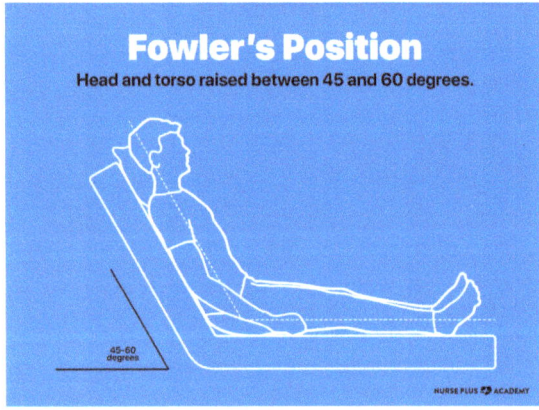
Illustration 9 https://nurse.plus

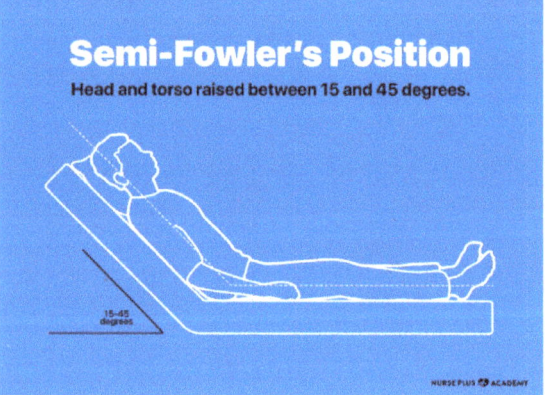
Illustration 8 https://nurse.plus/

Open airway maneuvers

- Head tilt – Chin lift:
    - Step 1: Place a hand on the infant or child's forehead, gently tilt the head back into the correct position:
        - Children: Sniffing
        - Infants: Neutral

- Step 2: Preform a chin lift by placing fingers under the chin, lifting gently upwards, without pressing on the soft tissue below the mandible

Head Tilt- Chin Lift

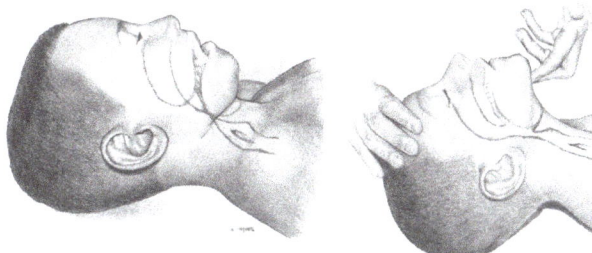
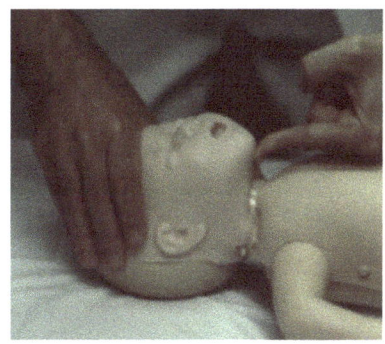

Illustration 10 Head tilt- Chin lift in neutral position

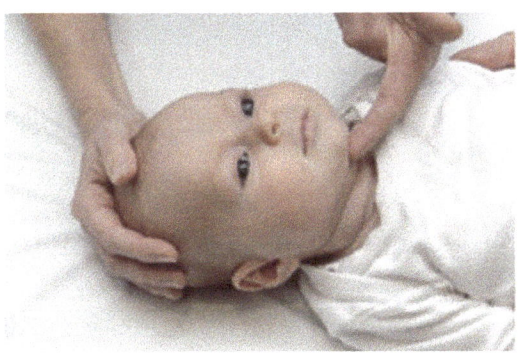
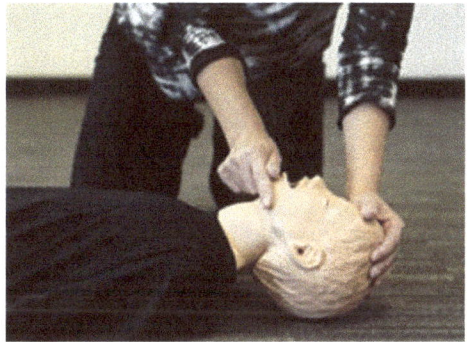

Illustration 11 Head tilt- Chin lift in neutral and sniffing position

- Head tilt – Chin lift is contraindicated if there is concern of possible spinal injury. In these cases, a jaw thrust manoeuvre is recommended.

- Jaw Thrust:
    - Place fingers behind the angles of the mandible and push anteriorly towards the tip of the nose

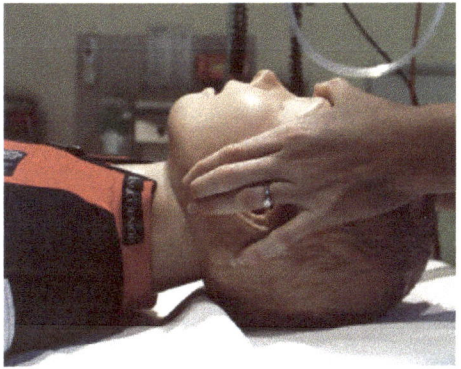
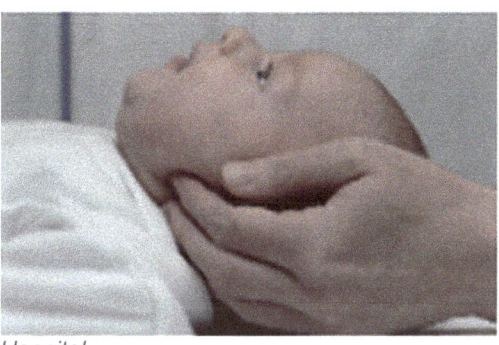

Illustration 12 Jaw thrust, The Royal Children´s Hospital

Oropharyngeal airway

- To keep the tongue from falling back and obstructing the airway.
- Size: distance from the central incisors to the angle of the jaw.

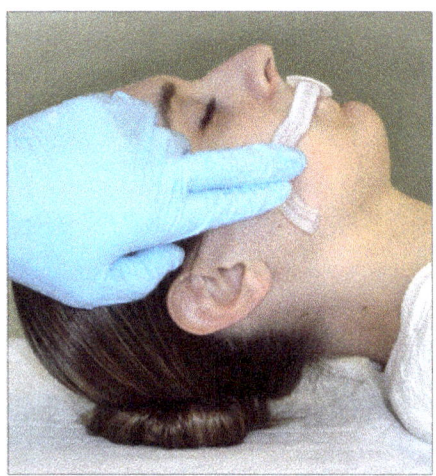

Illustration 13 Oropharyngela airway sizing, Uptodate, 2020

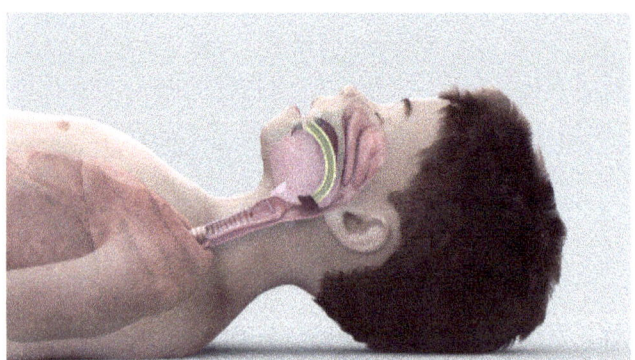

1: OPA proper size, AHA, 2020

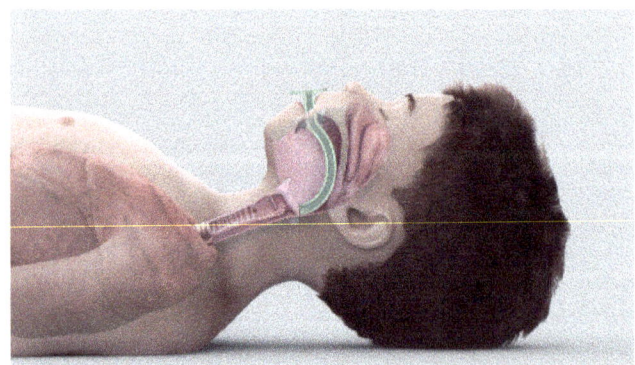

2: OPA too large (Will obstruct the airway by pushing the epiglotis down), AHA, 2020

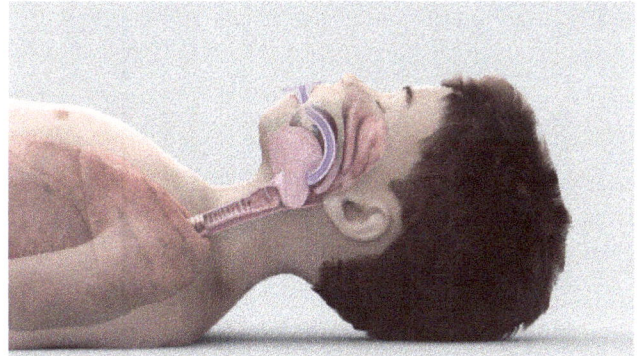

3: OPA too small (Will worsen airway obstruction by pushing the tongue into the back of the throat), AHA, 2020

Endotracheal tube (ETT)

- Endotracheal tube: The formula for estimation of a cuffed endotracheal tube size is:

    - **Uncuffed endotracheal tube size** (mm i.d.) = (age in years/4)+4
    - **Cuffed endotracheal tube size** (mm i.d.) = (age in years/4)+3.5
        - Typical cuffed inflation pressure should be <20 to 25 cm H_2O.

- Distance lip-tip (cm): ETT number (mm) x 3

- Example:
    - Child 8 years old:
    - Cuffed ETT → (age in years/4)+3.5 = (8/4)+ 3,5
        - Cuffed ETT number 5,5 mm (8/4)+ 3,5
        - Lip-tip (5,5 x3) = 17-18 cm

Pediatric Color-Coded Length-Based Resuscitation Tape

Zone	3 kg <3 mos	4 kg <3 mos	5 kg <3 mos	Pink 6–7 kg 3–5 mos	Red 8–9 kg 6–11 mos	Purple 10–11 kg 12–24 mos	Yellow 12–14 kg 2 yrs	White 15–18 kg 3–4 yrs	Blue 19–23 kg 5–6 yrs	Orange 24–29 kg 7–9 yrs	Green 30–36 kg 10–11 yrs
ETT uncuffed (mm)	3.5	3.5	3.5	3.5	3.5	4.0	4.5	5.0	5.5	N/A	N/A
ETT cuffed (mm)	3.0	3.0	3.0	3.0	3.0	3.5	4.0	4.5	5.0	5.5	6.0
Lip-tip (cm)	9-9.5	9.5-10	10-10.5	10-10.5	10.5-11	11-12	12.5-13.5	14-15	15.5-16.5	17-18	18.5-19.5
Suction (F)	8	8	8	8	8	8	10	10	10	10	12
L-scope blade	1 straight	1 straight	1 straight	1 straight	1 straight	1-1.5 straight	2 straight/curved	2 straight/curved	2 straight/curved	2-3 straight/curved	2-3 straight/curved
Stylet	6 F	6 F	6 F	6 F	6 F	6 F	10 F	10 F	10 F	14 F	14 F
OPA (mm)	50	50	50	50	50	60	60	60	70	80	80
NPA (F)	14	14	14	14	14	18	20	22	24	26	26
Bag-mask device (minimum mL)	450	450	450	450	450	450	450	450-750	750-1000	750-1000	1000
ETCO$_2$ detector	Ped	Ped	Ped	Ped	Ped	Ped	Ped	Adult	Adult	Adult	Adult
LMA	1	1	1	1.5	1.5	2	2	2	2-2.5	2.5	3
Tidal volume (mL)	20-30	24-40	30-50	40-65	50-85	65-105	80-130	100-165	125-210	160-265	200-330
Frequency	20-25/min	20-25/min	20-25/min	20-25/min	20-25/min	15-25/min	15-25/min	15-25/min	12-20/min	12-20/min	12-20/min

Abbreviations: ETT, endotracheal tube; F, French; LMA, laryngeal mask airway; NPA, nasopharyngeal airway; OPA, oropharyngeal airway; Ped, pediatric.
Adapted from the Broselow-Luten System Point of Care Guide © 2020 Vyaire Medical, Inc.;

Illustration 14 Pediatric color-coded length-based resuscitation tape, AHA, 2020

Breathing

Assessment

- Respiratory rate and pattern
- Respiratory effort:
    - Nasal flaring
    - Retractions
    - Head bobbing
    - Seesaw respirations
    - Open mouth breathing, gasping, use of accessory muscles
    - Grunting
- Chest expansion and air movement
- Lung and airway sounds
- O_2 saturation by pulse oximetry

	Oxygenation status	Action
SaO2 95-100%	**Normal**	Routine care
SaO2 92-94%	Almost normal	Monitoring
Sat 90-92%	Hypoxemia (mild)	Monitoring Consider oxygen
SaO2 80-89%	Hypoxemia (moderate)	Monitoring Give oxygen! ABCD
SaO2 < 80%	Hypoxemia (severe)	Monitoring Give oxygen! ABCD
Goal when giving oxygen → SaO2 95-97%		

Recognizing respiratory problems

Summary: Recognizing Respiratory Problems Flowchart

Table 29 summarizes recognition and identification of respiratory problems. Note that this chart does not include all respiratory emergencies but instead provides key characteristics for a limited number of diseases.

Table 29. Recognizing Respiratory Problems Flowchart

PALS: Signs of respiratory problems					
Clinical signs		Upper airway obstruction	Lower airway obstruction	Lung tissue disease	Disordered control of breathing
Airway	Patency	Airway open and maintainable/not maintainable			
Breathing	Respiratory rate/effort	Increased			Variable
	Breath sounds	Stridor (typically inspiratory) Barking cough Hoarseness	Wheezing (typically expiratory) Prolonged expiratory phase	Grunting Crackles Decreased breath sounds	Normal
	Air movement	Decreased			Variable
Circulation	Heart rate	Tachycardia (early); bradycardia (late)			
	Skin	Pallor, cool skin (early); cyanosis (late)			
Disability	Level of consciousness	Anxiety, agitation (early); lethargy, unresponsiveness (late)			
Exposure	Temperature	Variable			
PALS: Identifying respiratory problems by severity					
Progression of respiratory distress to respiratory failure*					
Airway		Respiratory distress: open and maintainable Respiratory failure: not maintainable			
Breathing		Respiratory distress: tachypnea Respiratory failure: bradypnea to apnea			
		Respiratory distress: work of breathing (nasal flaring/retractions) Respiratory failure: increased effort progresses to decreased effort and then to apnea			
		Respiratory distress: good air movement Respiratory failure: poor to absent air movement			
Circulation		Respiratory distress: tachycardia Respiratory failure: bradycardia			
		Respiratory distress: pallor Respiratory failure: cyanosis			
Disability		Respiratory distress: anxiety, agitation Respiratory failure: lethargy to unresponsiveness			
Exposure		Variable temperature			

Illustration 15 Recognizing respiratory problems flowchart, AHA, 2020

Bag mask ventilation

- Choose the correct sized face mask: This is important as an ill-fitting mask will result in a poor seal, leading to ineffective ventilation.

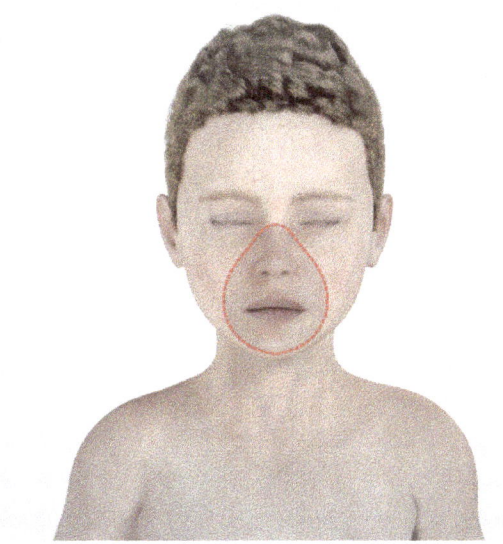

Illustration 16 Correct sized mask, AHA, 2020

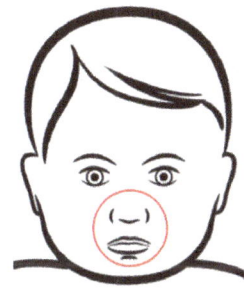

Correct Fit

A correctly fitted mask should sit on the bridge of the nose, cover the entire mouth and finish on the cleft of the chin. It should provide an air-tight seal.

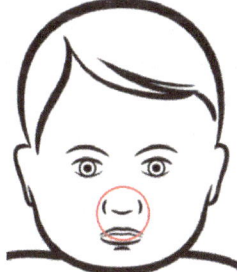

Too Small

A mask that is too small will not fully cover the nose and mouth.

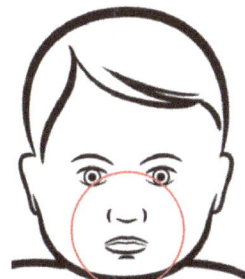

Too Big

A mask that is too big, may cover the eyes partially or extend over the chin.

An ill-fitting mask will result in a poor seal, leading to ineffective ventilation.

Illustration 17 Choosing correct sized face mask, Children´s Health Queensland Hospital and Health Service

- Bag mask ventilation technique:

Step 1: Using your non-dominant hand take your thumb and index finger and hold the mask with your fingers in the 'C' shape
Step 2: Use your other three fingers to make an 'E' shape, lifting the mandible. This helps to lift the tongue, thus assisting in opening the airway. Your little finger should be positioned at the angle of the jaw
Step3: Use your dominant hand on the self-inflating bag to deliver breaths.
Rhythm:
- Newborn 40 bpm
- Infant: 30 bpm
- Child: 20 bpm

Step 4: Observe the rise and fall of the chest for feedback on the adequacy of the seal

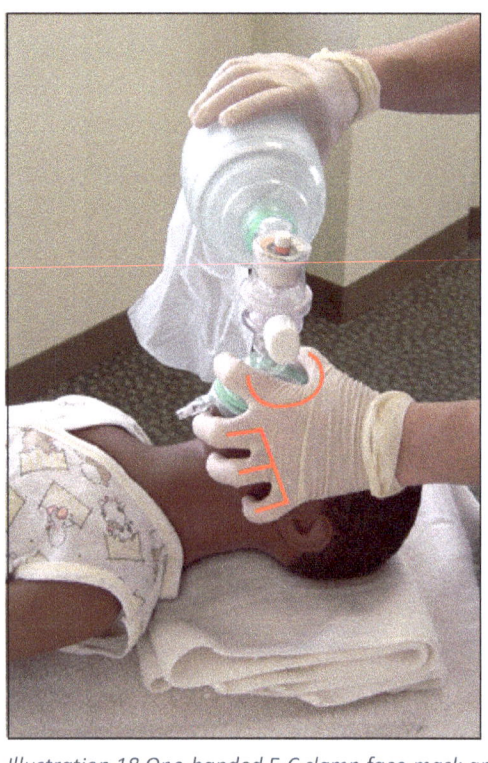
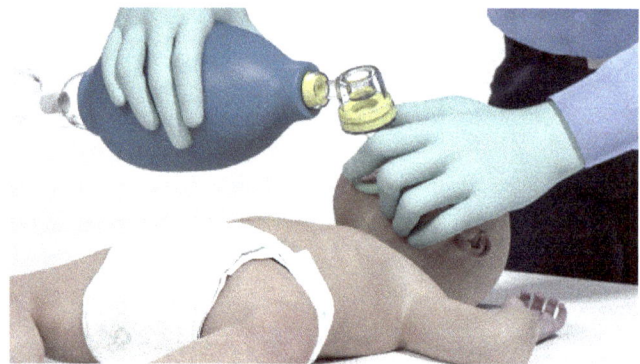

Illustration 18 One-handed E-C clamp face-mask application technique: 3 fingers lift the jaw (forming E) while thumb and index hold the mask to the mac, Uptodate 2022 & AHA 2020

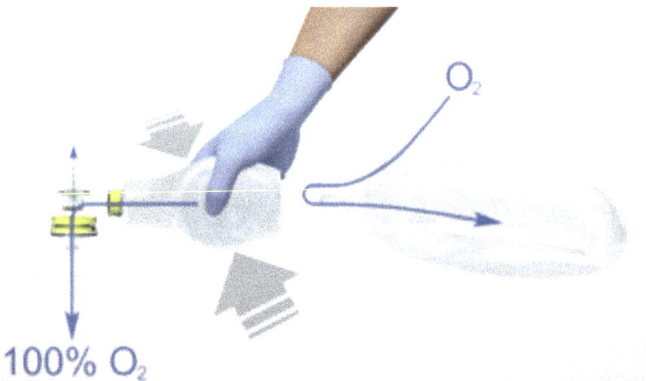

Respiratory failure: initial management

Table 30. Initial Management of Respiratory Distress or Failure

Evaluate	Interventions (as indicated)

Airway	• Support an open airway (allow child to assume position of comfort) or, if necessary, open the airway with
	  – Head tilt–chin lift
	  – Jaw thrust without head tilt if you suspect cervical spine injury. If this maneuver does not open the airway, use the head tilt–chin lift or jaw thrust with gentle head extension
	• Clear the airway if indicated (eg, suction nose and mouth, remove visualized foreign body).
	• Consider an oropharyngeal airway or nasopharyngeal airway to improve airway openness/patency.

Breathing	• Monitor O_2 saturation by pulse oximetry. • Provide O_2 (humidified if available). Use a high-concentration delivery device such as a nonrebreathing mask for treating severe respiratory distress or possible respiratory failure. • Administer inhaled medication (eg, albuterol, epinephrine) as needed. • Assist ventilation with bag-mask device and supplemental O_2 if needed. • Prepare for inserting an advanced airway if indicated.
Circulation	• Monitor heart rate, heart rhythm, and blood pressure. • Establish vascular access (for fluid therapy and medications) as indicated.

Illustration 19 Respiratory failures: initial management, AHA 2020

Respiratory emergencies flowchart

Summary: Managing Respiratory Emergencies Flowchart

The Managing Respiratory Emergencies Flowchart summarizes general management of respiratory emergencies and specific management by etiology (Table 36). This chart does not include all respiratory emergencies but provides key management strategies for a limited number of diseases.

Table 36. Managing Respiratory Emergencies Flowchart

Managing respiratory emergencies flowchart		
• Airway positioning • Suction as needed	• Oxygen • Pulse oximetry	• ECG monitor as indicated • BLS as indicated
Upper airway obstruction Specific management for selected conditions		
Croup	**Anaphylaxis**	**Aspiration foreign body**
• Nebulized epinephrine • Corticosteroids	• IM epinephrine (or autoinjector) • Albuterol • Antihistamines • Corticosteroids	• Allow position of comfort • Specialty consultation

Lower airway obstruction Specific management for selected conditions	
Bronchiolitis	**Asthma**
• Nasal suctioning • Consider bronchodilator trial	• Albuterol ± ipratropium • Corticosteroids • Magnesium sulfate • IM epinephrine (if severe) • Terbutaline
Lung tissue disease Specific management for selected conditions	
Pneumonia/pneumonitis Infectious, chemical, aspiration	**Pulmonary edema** Cardiogenic or noncardiogenic (ARDS)
• Albuterol • Antibiotics (as indicated) • Consider noninvasive or invasive ventilatory support with PEEP	• Consider noninvasive or invasive ventilatory support with PEEP • Consider vasoactive support • Consider diuretic

Disordered control of breathing Specific management for selected conditions		
Increased ICP	**Poisoning/overdose**	**Neuromuscular disease**
• Avoid hypoxemia • Avoid hypercarbia • Avoid hyperthermia • Avoid hypotension	• Antidote (if available) • Contact poison control	• Consider noninvasive or invasive ventilatory support

Illustration 20 Managing respiratory emergencies flowchart, AHA 2020

Circulation

Assess Circulation

- Heart rate and rhythm
- Pulses (both peripheral and central)
- Capillary refill time (normal < 2 seconds)
- Skin color and temperature
- Blood pressure
- Urine output
- Level of consciousness

- If HR < 60/min with signs of cardiopulmonary compromise → Start chest compressions (page 28)

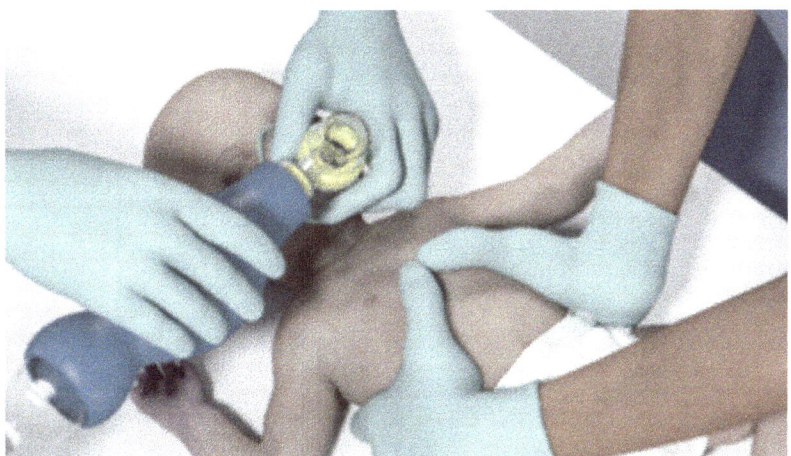

Illustration 21 Cardiopulmonary resuscitation, AHA, 2020

Recognizing shock

- Signs and symptoms of shock:
    - Tachycardia
    - Cold shock
        - Capillary refill > 2 seconds
        - ↓ Pulses
        - Discrepancy central vs. Distal pulses
    - Warm shock
        - Brisk capillary refill
        - Bounding peripheral pulses
        - Widened pulse pressure
    - ↓ Mental status
    - ↓ urine output
    - Metabolic acidosis (lactic)
    - Tachypnea
    - Hypotension (late sign)

Shock management

Managing Shock Flowchart

Table 55 summarizes general management of shock and specific management by etiology.

Table 55. Managing Shock Flowchart

Managing shock flowchart	
• Oxygen • Pulse oximetry • ECG monitor	• IV/IO access • BLS as indicated • Point-of-care glucose testing

Hypovolemic shock: Specific management for selected conditions	
Nonhemorrhagic	Hemorrhagic
• 20 mL/kg NS/LR bolus, repeat as needed • Consider colloid	• Control external bleeding • 20 mL/kg NS/LR bolus, repeat 2 or 3x as needed • Transfuse PRBCs as indicated

Distributive shock: Specific management for selected conditions		
Septic	Anaphylactic	Neurogenic
Management algorithm: • Septic Shock	• IM epinephrine (or autoinjector) • Fluid boluses (10-20 mL/kg NS/LR) • Albuterol • Antihistamines, corticosteroids • Epinephrine infusion	• 20 mL/kg NS/LR bolus, repeat PRN • Vasopressor

Cardiogenic shock: Specific management for selected conditions	
Bradyarrhythmia/tachyarrhythmia	Other (eg, CHD, myocarditis, cardiomyopathy, poisoning)
Management algorithms: • Bradycardia • Tachycardia	• 5 to 10 mL/kg NS/LR bolus, repeat PRN • Inotropic and/or vasoactive infusion • Consider expert consultation • Antidote for poisoning

Obstructive shock:

Specific management for selected conditions			
Ductal-dependent (LV outflow obstruction)	**Tension pneumothorax**	**Cardiac tamponade**	**Pulmonary embolism**
• Prostaglandin E1 • Expert consultation	• Needle decompression • Tube thoracostomy	• Pericardiocentesis • 20 mL/kg NS/LR bolus	• 20 mL/kg NS/LR bolus, repeat PRN • Consider thrombolytics, anticoagulants • Expert consultation

Illustration 22 Managing shock flowchart, AHA, 2020.

Pediatric septic Shock algorithm

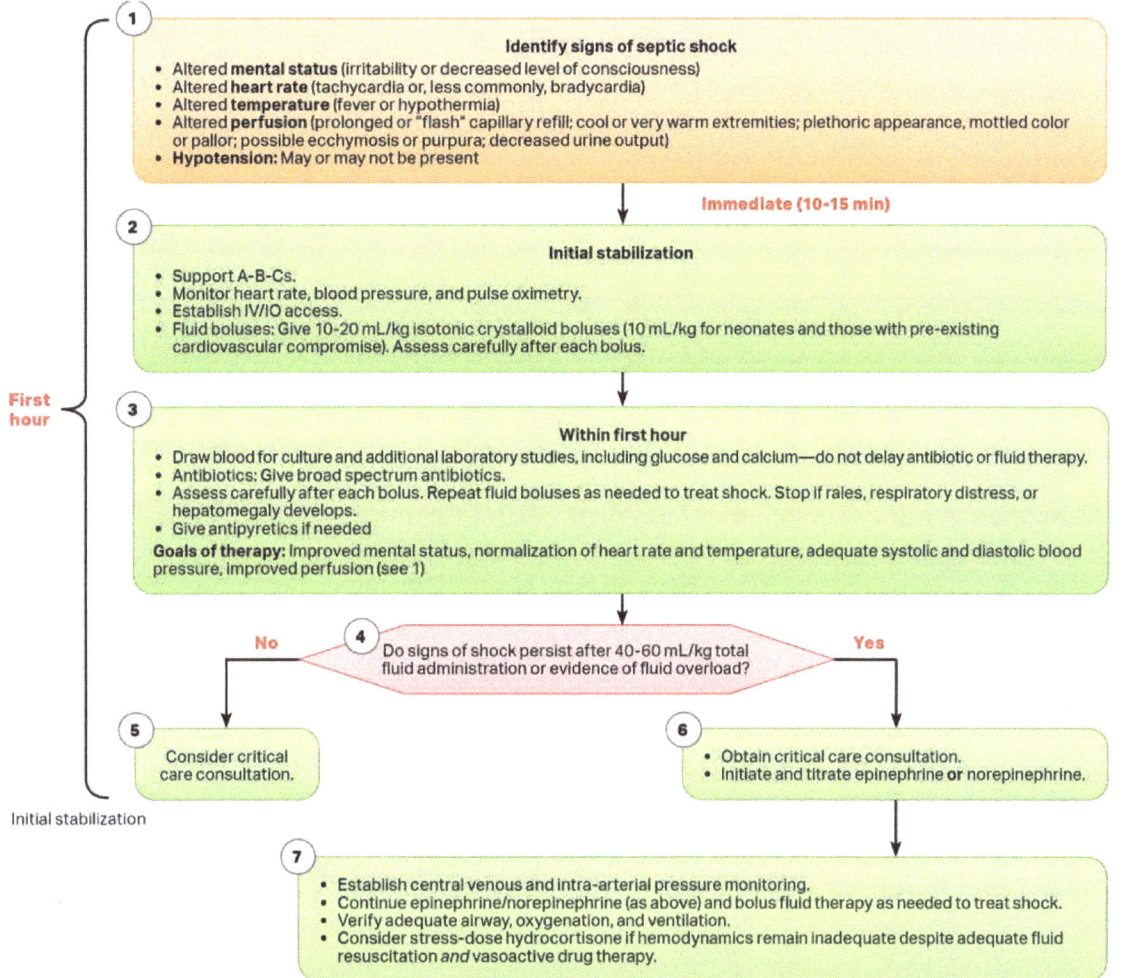

Illustration 23 Illustration 1 Pediatric Septic Shock Algorithm, AHA 2020.

Pediatric cardiac arrest algorithm

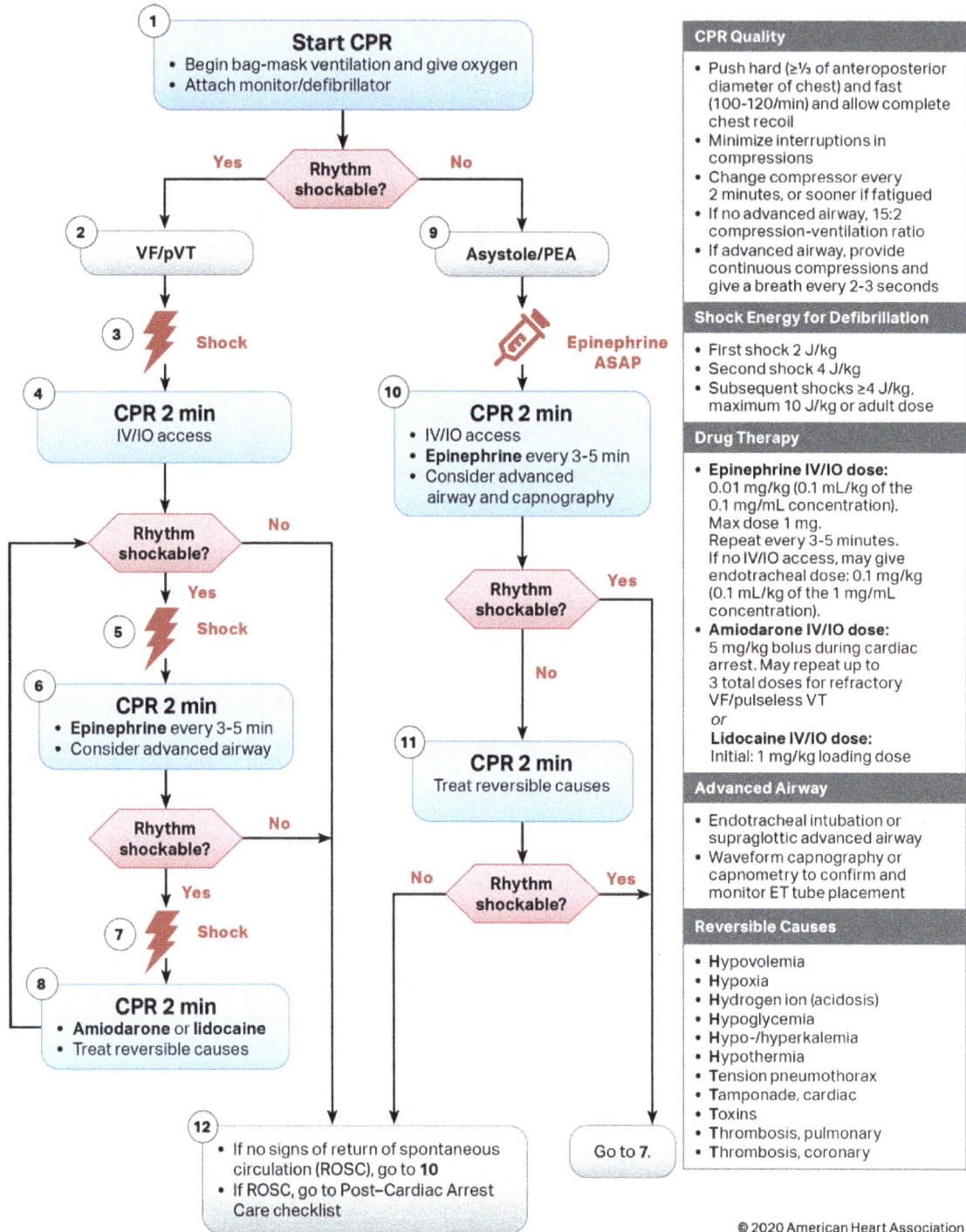

Illustration 24 Pediatric cardiac arrest algorithm. AHA, 2020.

Fluid therapy

Assessment

- Weight: all children on IV fluids should be weighed at the start of treatment and at least daily
- Evaluate hydration status: Weight, Pulse, BP, capillary refill, neurological status, urine output
- Evaluate signs of fluid overload in children receiving IV fluids (edema: periorbital, genital, sacral, peripheral, lungs)
- The severity of dehydration is measured as the acute weight loss as a % of pre-illness weight:
    o
- Pre-illness weight is often not available: use table

Finding	Mild (3 to 5%)	Moderate (6 to 9%)	Severe (≥10%)
Pulse	Full, normal rate	Rapid*	Rapid* and weak **or** absent
Systolic pressure	Normal	Normal to low	Low
Respirations	Normal	Deep, rate may be increased	Deep, tachypnea **or** decreased to absent
Buccal mucosa	Tacky or slightly dry	Dry	Parched
Anterior fontanelle	Normal	Sunken	Markedly sunken
Eyes	Normal	Sunken	Markedly sunken
Tears (in infants)	Present	Decreased	Absent
Skin turgor	Normal	Reduced	Tenting
Skin temperature and appearance	Normal	Cool	Cool, mottled, acrocyanosis
Urine output	Normal or mildly reduced	Markedly reduced	Anuria
Systemic signs	Increased thirst	Listlessness, irritability	Grunting, lethargy, coma

Illustration 25 Uptodate, 2022.

Fluid therapy: Why? What? How much?

- Why?
    o Shock or circulatory dysfunction → Fluid resuscitation
    o Unable to eat → Maintenance
    o Dehydration → Rehydration

- What?
    o Resuscitation: isotonic fluids (Na similar to plasma). No glucose!
    o Maintenance: isotonic fluid + Glucose + KCl
        ▪ < 3 months or < 5 kg:

-
  -
    -
      - Isotonic fluid (Saline 0,9%) + 10% glucose
    - \> 3 months:
      - Isotonic fluid (Saline 0,9%) + 5% glucose
    - How to prepare Glucosaline:
      - 500 ml of Saline 0,9% + 100 ml glucose 50% → Glucosaline 10-0,9% (for < 3 m)
      - 500 ml of Saline 0,9% + 50 ml glucose 50% → Glucosaline 5-0,9% (for > 3 m)
  - Rehydration: isotonic fluids + Glucose + KCl

- How much?
  - Resuscitation: 10-20 ml/kg
  - Maintenance: 4-3-2 rule +/- restriction*
  - Rehydration: Maintenance + deficit + ongoing losses
  - Renal failure: insensible losses + ongoing losses
  - *Restriction: 2/3 every sick child. Very critically ill 50% restriction
  - **Insensible losses: 300-400 ml/m2

- Resuscitation:
  - 10-20 ml/kg
  - Isotonic solutions:
    - 0,9% Normal Saline
    - Ringer´s Lactate
    - Hartmann´s
    - Plasma-Lyte
- Maintenance:

Weight (kg)	Full maintenance (ml/h) Well child	2/3 maintenance (ml/h) Sick child (unless dehydrated)
3	12	8
4	17	11
5	20	13
8	30	20
10	40	27
15	50	33
20	60	40
25	65	43
30	70	46
35	75	50
40	80	53
45	85	57
50	90	60
55	95	63
>60	100	67

- Rehydration:
    - First: calculate the degree of dehydration
    - Total fluids requirement = replacement of deficit + maintenance + replacement of ongoing losses
        - Maintenance = see table
        - Fluid deficit formula:
            - Deficit = (pre-illness weight (kg) – current weight) x 1000
            - If pre-illness weight not known: weight (kg) x 10 x % dehydration
    - Replace deficit over 24-28 hours
        - Dehydration < 5%: replace deficit in 24 hours
        - Dehydration > 5%: replace deficit more slowly: 48 hours
        - Serial clinical assessment of hydration status must be made at regular intervals
    - Ongoing losses: ongoing losses should be measured and replaced each 4 hours

- Hypoglycemia:
    - Glucose 0,2 g/kg IV
        - = 2 ml/kg of Glucose 10%
        - = 0,5 ml/kg of Glucose 50%

Fluid therapy flowchart

Situation	What	Type of fluid	Fluid	How much?
Shock	Resuscitation	Isotonic No glucose!	Saline 0,9%	20 ml/kg
Unable to eat < 3 months	Maintenance	Isotonic + 10% glucose + KCl	Glucosaline 10-0,9%*	See fluid calculator ml/h
Unable to eat > 3 months	Maintenance	Isotonic + 5% glucose + KCl	Glucosaline 5-0,9%**	See fluid calculator ml/h
Dehydration	Rehydration	Isotonic + 5% glucose + KCl	Glucosaline 5-0,9%**	See fluid calculator ml/h (24 h) + deficit (weight (kg) x 10 x % dehydration)
Hypoglycemia Glucose < 60 mg/dl (2,8 mmol/l)		Glucose	Glucose 10%	2 ml/kg
			Glucose 50%	0,5 ml/kg

* Glucosaline 10-0,9% = 500 ml of Saline 0,9% + 100 ml glucose 50%
** Glucosaline 5-0,9% = 500 ml of Saline 0,9% + 50 ml glucose 50%

Maintenance fluid calculator

Weight (kg)	Full maintenance (ml/h) Well child	2/3 maintenance (ml/h) Sick child (unless dehydrated)
3	12	8
4	17	11
5	20	13
8	30	20
10	40	27
15	50	33
20	60	40
25	65	43
30	70	46
35	75	50
40	80	53
45	85	57
50	90	60
55	95	63
>60	100	67

Newborn fluid therapy

	Type of fluid	How much?
Day 1 of life	Glucose 10%	60 ml/kg/day
Day 2 of life	Glucose of 10%	80 ml/kg/day
Day 3 of life	Glucosaline 10-0,9%*+ ClK	100 ml/kg/day
> 3 days of life	Glucosaline 10-0,9%* + ClK	120 ml/kg/day
Glucosaline* 10-0,9% = 500 ml of Saline 0,9% + 100 ml glucose 50%		

Normal glucose levels:

- 24 hours of life: 45-125 mg/dl (2,5- 6,9 mmol/l)
- 24-48 hours of life: 50 mg/dl (2,8-6,9 mmol/l)
- \> 48 hours- 1 week: 60 mg/dl (3,3-6,9 mmol/l)
- \> 1 week of life: 70-100 mg/dl (3,9-5,6 mmol/l)

Disability

Assess disability

- AVPU Pediatric Response Scale (*A*lert, Responsive to *V*oice, Responsive to *P*ain, *U*nresponsive)
- Glasgow Coma Scale (GCS)
- Pupil response to light
- Blood glucose test

Glasgow coma scale

Glasgow Coma Scale*

Score	Child	Infant
Eye opening		
4	Spontaneously	Spontaneously
3	To verbal command	To shout, speech
2	To pain	To pain
1	No response	No response
Best motor response		
6	Obeys commands	Spontaneous movements
5	Localizes pain	Withdraws to touch
4	Flexion-appropriate withdraw	Flexion-appropriate withdraw
3	Flexion-abnormal (decorticate rigidity)	Flexion-abnormal (decorticate rigidity)
2	Extension (decerebrate rigidity)	Extension (decerebrate rigidity)
1	No response	No response
Best verbal response		
5	Oriented and converses	Smiles, coos, and babbles
4	Disoriented, confused	Cries but is consolable
3	Inappropriate words	Persistent, inappropriate crying and/or screaming
2	Incomprehensible sounds	Moans, grunts to pain
1	No response	No response

Illustration 26 Glasgow coma scale, AHA, 2020

- Severity of head injury is categorized into 3 levels based on GCS score after initial resuscitation:
    - Mild head injury: GCS score 13 to 15
    - Moderate head injury: GCS score 9 to 12
    - Severe head injury: GCS score 3 to 8

Blood glucose test

- Normal:
- Hypoglycemia child < 60 mg/dl (3,3 mmol/l)
- Hypoglycemia newborn:
    - 24 hours of life: < 45 mg/dl (2,5 mmol/l)
    - 24-48 hours of life: < 50 mg/dl (2,8 mmol/l)
    - \> 48 hours- 1 week or older: < 60 mg/dl (3,3 mmol/l)

- If hypoglycemia: give glucose 0,2 g/kg:
    - Glucose 10%: 2 ml/kg or
    - Glucose 50%: 0,5 ml/kg

Abnormal pupil responses and possible causes

Abnormal pupil response	Possible cause
Pinpoint pupils	• Narcotic ingestion (eg, opioid)
Dilated pupils	• Predominant sympathetic autonomic activity • Sympathomimetic ingestion (eg, cocaine) • Anticholinergic ingestion (eg, local or systemic atropine) • Increased intracranial pressure
Unilaterally dilated pupils	• Inadvertent topical absorption of a breathing treatment (eg, ipratropium) • Dilating eye drops
Unilaterally dilated pupils with altered mental status	• Ipsilateral (same side) uncal herniation (lateral herniation of the temporal lobe, caused by increased intracranial pressure)

Illustration 27 Abnormal pupil responses, AHA, 2020

Seizures flowchart

Seizures	
0 min	ABCD: Continuous monitoring Support airway Provide Oxygen Support ventilation (BMV) if needed Obtain IV/IO access Check temperature Check glucose (< 60 mg/dl → Glucose 10% 2 ml/kg)
5 min	Fist-line agents: benzodiazepines
10 min	Repeat benzodiazepine (maximum 2 doses)
15 min	Second-line agent ICU
20 min	Alternative second-line agent
25 min	Third-line agent Airway management Support ventilation
First-line agents = benzodiazepines: - Midazolam: IV/IO/IM 0,15 mg/kg (max 10 mg) - Midazolam buccal: 0,3 mg/kg (max 10 mg) - Diazepam IV/IO: 0,3 mg/kg (max 10 mg) - Diazepam PR: 0,5 mg/kg (max 10 mg, not IM) - Side effects benzodiazepines: respiratory depression	
Second-line agents: - Phenobarbitone IV 20 mg/kg (max 1 g) administered over a minimum of 20 minutes. Doi not exceed 1 mg/kg/min to avoid respiratory and/or circulatory compromise. - Phenytoin IV 20 mg/kg (max 1,5 g) over a minimum of 20 minutes. Dilute 20 mg/ml. Stop infusion when seizure ceases. Side effects: arrhythmias, respiratory depression. - Levetiracetam IV 60 mg/kg (max 4,5 g) over 5 minutes. No side effects.	
Third-line agents: - Midazolam infusion 1 mcg/kg/min - Propofol 2,5 mg/kg IV/IO + infusion 1-3 mg/kg/h. Beware hypotension. - Thiopentone 2-5 mg/kg IV/IO + 1-4 mg/kg/h. Beware hypotension.	

Bibliography

.Pediatric Advanced Life Support, American Heart Association AHA, 2020.
.Clinical Practice Guidelines of The Royal Children´s Hospital Melbourne.
https://www.rch.org.au/clinicalguide/
.Paediatric intensive care. Oxford specialist handbooks in paediatrics, 2017.
.Uptodate 2022.
.Paediatric BASIC: Basic Assessment and Support in Paediatric Intensive Care. Bruce Lister, PICU. 3rd edition, April 2017.
.Pedscases: pediatric vital signs reference chart, The Hospital for Sick Children in Toronto, Canada.
.Nursing skill sheets, Queensland Paediatric Emergency care. Children´s Health Queensland Hospital and Health Service.

www.ingramcontent.com/pod-product-compliance
Lightning Source LLC
Chambersburg PA
CBHW050146180526
45172CB00012B/1323